Living Your Retirement Dreams and Growing Young in The Villages;

Florida's Friendliest and Healthiest Hometown

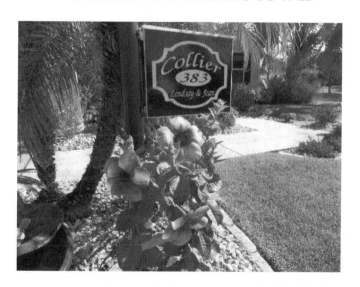

Lindsay Collier

Published by Create Space,

an Amazon company

ISBN - 13-978-1505481730

ISBN -10 1505481732

Table of Contents

Foreword

In the heart of Central Florida about 70 miles northwest from Orlando exists what is probably the biggest retirement community in the world called The Villages. My wife Jean and I bought a home here in the fall of 2005. Although we still go back to family in Rochester, New York for a good part of the summer, we are permanent residents of Florida and consider this our own little "paradise," It is a truly unique place unlike anything we've ever seen. When we decided we wanted to move to a warm climate we explored a few areas of Florida (mainly the Naples/Bonita Springs area), and on a trip back decided to drive up through Central Florida. We ended up stopping for lunch in Spanish Springs which was at that time the only downtown area of The Villages. I remember Jean looking at all the people happily driving around in their golf carts and saying, "These people are all so happy - they must be on something."

A few months later we came back on one of the visitation packages for a week and decided that this was where we wanted to make our home. And, voila, here we are. They call this **Florida's Friendliest Home Town** and it definitely lives up to its name. I'm writing this in part because it seems there is a lot of information lately that would have you believe that The Villages is a place full of sex-crazed old people popping Viagra pills and chasing each other around; and it is just not like that at all. It's funny how fast a little saucy information travels. In reality The Villages is chocked full of some of the nicest people you could ever meet. Hardy a week goes by without news of several 50 or 60 year wedding anniversaries and Villagers continually go out of their way to help each other out. It is an incredibly caring community! The voter turnout here is at 80% - the average Villager cares deeply about their community and their country. And, the range of talent among the folks here is just incredible! Also, The Villages has one of the lowest crime rates in the country.

The prevailing attitude is that of people who are here living out their retirement dreams. We sometimes refer to it as **God's Waiting Room**. There are **snowbirds** (just come down for the winter months), **snowflakes** (just go back for the northern summers), **heatbirds** (can't stand the heat and want to get out of the kitchen), and **frogs** (we are here till we croak). Some of the common sayings include, "It's just nice to be above ground." and, "It is what it is."

My purpose here is to create a sort of operating manual for those who live in The Villages and also to give those who are currently contemplating retirement an idea of what this community offers. In the EBook version there over 100 website links so that you can bounce between reading the text and the expanded information on the appropriate websites. In the paperback version those items which are underlined are generally the ones which have hyperlinks in the EBook. You may want to consider buying the Kindle version along with the paperback to take advantage of these links.

Amazon.con offers a free app for your Smartphone, IPAD, laptop, PC or other device that gives you a Kindle site so you can download and use Kindle versions. And there are many advantages such as the ability to directly connect to websites, underline, highlight, copy and paste, add bookmarks, change print size, and more. You can also easily arrange your books into various collections. Try it I think you'll like it!

I sincerely hope you enjoy it and would love to hear from you anytime with any comments, additions, additional words of wisdom, etc. You can reach me at **lindsaycollier@comcast.net.**

Lindsay Collier - Village of Tall Trees

Chapter 1

A Day in the Life of The Villages

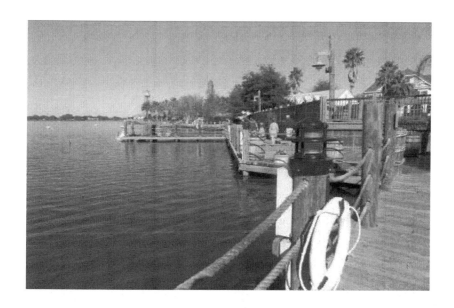

History of The Villages

Let's begin with a short history of The Villages which begin back in the 1970's. Wikopedia has an excellent and complete history if you would like to get into more detail. In the early 70's Harold Schwartz began development of a mobile home park called Orange Blossom Gardens in the northwest corner of Lake County. His stated goal from the beginning was to offer a millionaire's lifestyle on a retirement budget. Free golf was a part of the early vision. By the early 80's they had sold only about 400 units, and Mr. Schwartz decided to buy out his partner's share and bring his son, H. Gary Morse, on board in 1983.

Building on what some successful retirement communities like Del Webb's Sun City were doing by providing certain amenities to their residents as well as having diverse and nearby commercial development,

Mr. Morse began to significantly upgrade the development. As sales improved through the 80's, Schwartz began to buy large tracts of land in Marian and Sumter Counties. In 1992 it was officially named The Villages.

It has grown at a healthy and growing rate; and in the last few years, the growth has been phenomenal. The Villages now is one of the fastest growing communities in the United States (and probably the world). It spreads through 3 counties (Lake, Marion, and Sumter). Sumter county was once one the least developed and poorest counties in Florida and is now one of the most successful. At this point the property of the Villages covers over 32 square miles and some 23,000 acres. A recent purchase of land in the adjacent town of Fruitland Park has added to this. Baby boomers have contributed a great deal to the recent growth.

H. Gary Morse passed away in 2014, and his family have vowed to continue his legacy. The Morse family lives on 2,754 acres - 4.3 square miles off CR 466 in the heart of The Villages.

Layout of The Villages

Florida for the most part is as flat as a pancake. The Villages is about an hour northwest from Orlando's airport and about 30 miles south of Ocala. Much of it is in what I would call 'rolling hills country' and much more scenic than other parts of the state. Its location in Central Florida allows access to either the ocean front or the gulf in a little over an hour. The nearest cities are Leesburg and Ocala which offer all the amenities that are usually found in small cities. But one could easily survive and thrive for the most part without ever leaving The Villages. And most everything you need is within golf car range. There are over 100 miles of golf trails and access to pretty much all the commercial amenities you'll ever need.

The Villages covers 26,000 acres or 32 square miles in three counties, Lake, Marion, and Sumter. It is about 8.5 miles east to west and 15 miles north to south. Projected population in 2016 is 105,000. Here's how the population has grown in the past few years:

- 1992 was 11,000

- 2000 was 21,000

- 2006 was 60,000

- 2010 was 80,000

- 2014 is about 100,000

- Annual growth is about 4,500

Need to go to the supermarket (Publix, Winn Dixie, Wal-Mart, Fresh Market are the main ones here)? Just jump in your golf cart with your grocery bag attachment and go for it. If you need to go to Target, Staples, CVS, Walgreens, Bed Bath and Beyond, Best Buy, Kohl's, Beal's or dozens of other stores, it's same thing. And whatever your culinary desire might be there are dozens of restaurants within a short golf cart drive.

I'm sure there is no place in the world that has anywhere near the concentration of golf carts. Golf carts are the vehicle of choice for many residents. There are over 50,000 golf carts here, many of which are customized to owners' specs. Yamaha, EZGo, ClubCar, ParCar, and Star are the common brands. There is almost no place you can't get to in your cart as a resident. A series of golf cart trails include a number of tunnels to get you to all the shopping you will ever need. All the medical facilities you need are also golf cart accessible.

And I am sure there is no other place in the world with the number and variety of customized golf carts. There are '57 Chevys, Mustangs, Escalades, Porsches, roadsters and lots of Yesteryear designs. There are some set up as fire trucks, UPS delivery trucks, police cars and more. There are even a couple of custom semis that are quite amazing, complete with twin stacks and dual tandem wheels. And in 2005 the Guinness Book of Records was set for the longest golf cart parade with 3391 carts!

The Villages has 3 downtown areas, **Spanish Springs**, **Lake Sumter Landing**, and the newest, **Brownwood**. Each of these squares has a variety of shops and restaurants and an entertainment area where there is music and dancing every night of the year from 5 - 9pm. And, of course, each has several libation centers which offer a happy hour at various times. Speaking of happy hour, most restaurants in the area offer happy hours, some which last all day. Villagers love their happy hours. Cheers!

Spanish Springs is the oldest downtown area. It is done in a Spanish motif which is quite attractive. Until recently one of the focal points was The Church on the Square. It functioned as a non-denominational church as well as a forum for some wonderful entertainment and was the most attractive structure there.

2014-15 saw the expansion of the original structure into the Sharon Morse Center for Performing Arts (commonly referred to as "The Sharon") which opened in April 2015. This a state-of-the-art facility which promises to be a very exciting venue for future events and can accommodate over 1200 people.

Lake Sumter Landing was completed around 2005 and has somewhat of a Key West and New England appeal. It is a very busy area with some of the best shops and restaurants in the area. It is located adjacent to man-made Lake Sumter and affords great views and sunsets. Close to it is a place called Sunset Landing with a small golf cart park that is situated to give the best view of sunset. People gather there evenings to watch the sun set. We were there one night with an old Navy guy, and at sunset he went down to the water and played Taps. It was a tear jerking experience.

Brownwood is the latest which was just opened in 2013. It is designed as an old time Florida cattle town and is quite something to behold. The process of building Brownwood was truly amazing. New structures such as the three water towers were built, and then artists painted them to look like they were 100 years old.

Each of the squares has an entertainment pavilion as well as a multi-screen theater which is state of the art and very comfortable. There is entertainment every night of the year from 5-9 p.m. Special events such as St Patrick's Day, Oktoberfest, Italian fest, Mardi Gras, and others are celebrated seasonally. Each has a large and beautifully lit Christmas Tree during the holidays and a special tree lighting ceremony. Each Christmas there is also a special parade as well at the Polo Grounds.

One of the most interesting features of the squares are the cameras which are active 24 hours a day that can be accessed by anyone using the website, Villages Live Cameras. You can check to see how busy it is before you go there or perhaps invite your friends up north to check out your new pair of shorts as they huddle by their fireplaces.

Where do Villagers come from?

Most folks in The Villages are from the US but there are also sizeable groups of Canadians, Brits, Germans, Icelanders, and more. It turns out that the largest number of folks come to The Villages from other parts of Florida. Virtually all states are represented here and the following is the 2015 count of each state in descending order.

New York - 9509

Pennsylvania - 5601

Ohio - 5005

Michigan - 4798

Illinois - 3823

Wisconsin - 3039

Massachusetts - 3031

Virginia - 2338

Maryland - 2336

Connecticut - 2196

Indiana - 2149

Georgia - 1354

Minnesota - 1338

New Hampshire - 1206

North Carolina - 1075

California - 962

Missouri - 899

Rhode Island - 771

Maine - 770

Tennessee - 740

Kentucky - 669

Iowa - 651

Delaware - 466

Colorado - 449

West Virginia - 417

South Caralina - 405

Vermont - 399

Washington - 372

Alabama - 283

Kansas - 274

Nevada - 128

Arkansas - 123

Oregon - 116

Mississippi - 107

Oklahoma - 103

All other states have less than 100 people here.

Homes in The Villages

Homes in The Villages range from less than $100k to over $2 million dollars. The so called "historic section" which is east of route 441, contains a number of doublewides and prefabs is where you will find the least expensive homes. There is a movement under way now to buy up some of these older homes, tear them down, and build upgrades. The variety of homes includes patio villas, courtyard villas, ranch homes, designer homes, and premier homes. Most of the new homes in the southern section (south of route 466A) are well over the $250,000 mark. There are virtually all one-story homes with just a few exceptions, and don't expect a basement. This is Florida. I do miss that nice , musty cellar smell I've known for years.

It is well worth becoming a home owner in Florida since every person who owns and resides on real property in Florida on January 1 and makes the property his or her permanent residence is eligible to receive a homestead exemption up to $50,000. The first $25,000 applies to all property taxes, including school district taxes.

Each village has its own swimming pool, mail pickup area, and shuffle ball, bocce, and horse shoe courts. Some of the larger villages have recreation halls which have kitchen facilities, meeting areas, and billiards rooms. Swimming pools are abundant with some being designated as family pools, where grandchildren and other guests under 30 years old are welcome; and some as neighborhood adult pools, for residents and guests over 30. There are also several sport pools for organized swimming events (water exercise programs, laps, water volley ball, etc.). And several of the champion golf courses have their own pools, but you must be a priority member to use them.

Speaking of guests, residents are required to get guest passes for family and friends who are visiting if they would like to use any of the facilities such as pools, recreation halls or golf.

The Economy in the Villages

Recession - What recession? You hear that a lot in The Villages, and for good reason. Even in less than good times, the economy of The Villages keeps plugging along. There are about 17,000 paid employees in the Villages Metropolitan Statistical area according to the U.S. Census Bureau. Somewhere around 2,500 of these are in the construction business. About 2,600 are in food service and accommodation, 3,000 in health care, and 3,100 in retail trade. The unemployment rate in Sumter County is a full percentage below the national average.

Navigating The Villages

At first blush, navigating around the Villages may seem like a daunting task. But it's actually quite easy and quick to learn. Development has taken place from north to south. The so-called historic district is at the northeastern end in Lake County east of Route 441/27. West of 441 lies Spanish Springs, the first downtown area built in The Villages. South of Spanish Springs are the early villages which were built up through the 90's. As you proceed south there are three east/west roads, routes 466, 466A, and 44 that quite nicely encapsulate villages that have been more recently built. Rout 44 is the southern end of The Villages. Two major roads, Buena Vista and Morse Boulevard, cut north and south through The Villages. There are about 50 roundabouts in The Villages.

Getting around by golf cart has a few challenges at first but as long as you know the general layout and the main roads, it gets easier. There is also a Golf GPS App now available for your Smartphone (both Apple and Android) that can be very useful. It's called **The Villages GPS** and sells for $4.99. It comes pre-programmed with golf courses, town squares, restaurants, recreation centers, neighborhood villages, shopping, pools, and more

HELP! I'm Building and I Can't Stop.

The rate of expansion in The Villages is truly remarkable. The landscape seems to change almost on a daily basis. At one point they were talking about the build out ending at just north of Route 44 in the town of Wildwood. In 2014 and 2015 more land was purchased and three new parcels were announced. The largest of these extends into the town of Fruitland Park. If this remains a single village it will be the largest with 2048 homes and bring the total number of villages to 89!

There is a smaller parcel in the planning at the northern end of The Villages in Marian County. This will provide 2-300 new homes and villas.

Postal Services

It's hard to believe, but there are no Post Offices in The Villages. My wife and I go back to the Rochester, NY area for a few months in the summer and stay in a town that has about 1000 residents at the most (along with 5000 cows). This town has its own Post Office and The Villages with 100,000 people doesn't. Figure that one out! There are PO's in the surrounding communities most of which are quite inadequate to serve the number of people in the area - especially during the holidays.

Access to Airports

Orlando International Airport (MCO) and Orlando Sanford International (SFB) airports are about a one hour drive; Tampa International Airport (TPA) is about an hour and twenty minutes. The Villages has a shuttle to the Orlando airport five times a day from both Sumter Landing and Spanish Springs..

Villages Media

The Villages has all its own media. The Villages Daily Sun is, in my opinion, one of the best and most enjoyable newspapers ever. There is a lot of local news and sports coverage, and the coverage of national and worldly events is superb. It definitely leans toward conservative, but The Villages has a very high concentration of conservatives. They also have a free app that can be downloaded to your smart phone, IPad and most other similar devices. This is a great way to keep in touch with what's happening in The Villages - especially when traveling or when spending your summers in another location. You can read the stories in the daily paper, get breaking news, see what is going on at the Town Squares (entertainment and movies), check the Yellow Pages, see the weather, and even see a streaming video of the local Daily Sun News Show.

Once per month The Villages Magazine is delivered along with the newspaper. This is very well done and very tasteful reading. It is also available as a free App for your Kindle, Nook, or other eBook device.

Each Thursday the Recreation News is included with the newspaper. This is a summary of weekly events at recreation centers and club events. And on Saturday there a very nice addition called **The Mix** which focuses on news from neighbors in your area.

WVLG - 640 AM is The Villages radio station and always has a great selection of music along with news. There are several times in the week that they play lots of oldies which we Villagers of course love to hear; and there is Fox News coverage on the hour. It is piped into each of the squares as well. **TV 2 is** The Villages TV station and carries news that just focuses on local activities. And, as mentioned before, you can access the local news loop with the free app from the Daily Sun.

A relatively new independent site for news in The Villages can be found at Villages-News.com. This can be set up to arrive in your email daily for those who want to keep up with the latest.

Governing and Advocacy Groups in The Villages

Here's where it can get a little confusing. The Villages has three organizations that look out for the development and needs of residents:

The Villages Homeowners Association (VHA)

This association membership is somewhere in the vicinity of 25,000 and turns 23 years old in 2015. It's first project was a petition drive requesting approval for construction of a golf cart bridge over US 441/27. The mission of the VHA is to preserve and enhance the values of homes and The Villages' lifestyle. Their vision is to maintain The Villages as the premier 55-plus community in the world — featuring the finest amenities, homes, retail and commercial businesses, medical and professional services, as well as the best educational, cultural, recreational and entertainment opportunities. The fee for joining is $15 for 2 years or $60 for lifetime (per household). Once a month, a small newspaper called The Villages Voice is delivered to each home in The Villages along with the Daily Sun. The Villages is separated into 11 development districts including the latest and last which includes the parcel being developed in the town of Fruitland Park in 2014-2015. Each Village has locale representatives. They also sponsor New Resident's Night twice a month at the Colony Cottage Recreation Center to welcome and orient new residents.

Villages Community Development (VCD)

This organization has the mission to provide responsible and accountable public service that enhances and sustains the community and to provide and preserve its lifestyle. They oversee services such as guest passes, utility fees, recreation centers, ID cards, fitness centers, facility rental, and more. Guests over 1 year old should have guest passes, which are available at no cost through their website. The guest pass is needed to use any of the amenities such as golf, swimming pools, recreation centers or Katie Belles, a "resident only" restaurant/music hall.

A key area of VCD is the overseeing of the **Community Watch program**. This is not a law enforcement agency, but it works closely with the local Sheriff's Departments. They conduct roving patrols throughout The Villages and also staff all the gates. They have a home watch service as well as providing a watch while a resident is away. And they also have an Adult Watch Program for residents that live alone or residents with a partner who needs someone to give them a call to see if they are in good standing.

Property Owners Association (POA)

Founded in 1975 as the original homeowner's association, The Property Owners' Association of the Villages is an independent organization devoted to the home ownership needs and interests of the residents of The Villages. The Vision/Objective of the POA is to make The Villages an even better place in which to live, where Residents' Rights are respected, and local government is responsive to the needs and interests of residents. It has no tie or obligations to the developer that might compromise its advocacy of residents' rights.

Recreation Centers

There are currently 9 Regional Recreation Centers and 22 Recreation Centers. Regional Centers offer large and small (adjustable) meeting rooms and are the venue for many club meetings and activities. Each one has a dance hall size room for large meetings and an outside pavilion for outdoor events. The more numerous recreation centers are smaller, and have smaller meeting rooms, kitchen facilities, and very nice billiard rooms. A Villages or guest ID is required to use these facilities, although I believe outside groups can rent them as available. These buildings are very tastefully decorated along the lines of various themes.

At the time of this writing the latest Regional Recreation Center is Eisenhower which is dedicated to veterans and contains an absolutely remarkable collection of memorabilia from wars, much of it contributed by offspring of veterans who are residents here.

Here are the current recreation centers:

Regional Centers:

- Paradise

- La Hacienda

- Savannah

- Mulberry Grove

- Laurel Manor

- Lake Miona

- Colony Cottage

- Seabreeze

- Eisenhower

- Rohan

Village Recreation Centers:

- Silver lake

- Southside

- Chula Vista

- Tierra Del Sol

- Saddlebrook

- El Santiago

- Chatham

- Bridgeport

- Churchill

- Pimlico

- Bacall

- Canal Street

- Coconut Cove

- Odell

- Truman

- Alameda

- Fish Hawk

- Hibiscus

- Sterling Heights

- Big Cypress

- Bradenton

- Captiva

- Manatee

- Moyer

All recreations centers are Wi-Fi capable, and the Savannah Center has a computer room for residents. All Recreational Centers also have mobile, well-stocked first aid kits with band aids, gauze bandages, tape, and ice packs.

Parks in The Villages

As of 2014, The Villages contains 17 parks within its property:

- o Ashland Park
- o Boone Park
- o Brinson-Perry Dog Park
- o Golfview Lake
- o Lake Miona Fitness Trail
- o Lake Mira Mar
- o Live Oaks Park
- o Mulberry Dog Park
- o Paradise Dog Park
- o Paradise Lake

- Schwartz Park

- Springdale Fitness Trail

- Springdale Walking Trail

- Sunset Park

- Veteran's Memorial Park

- Wilkerson Creek and Children's Playground Center

Their locations can be found in the Recreation News.

Weather in The Villages

For a good part of the year the weather is just spectacular. Coming from Rochester, New York that is easy for me to say. October, November, March, and April are the best months. December, January, and February are also very nice months, although there are often some cold spells when the evenings can drop below freezing. Hard freezes are not uncommon during these months. But the daytime temperatures almost always work their way about to comfortable levels. Mid May through mid September can be uncomfortably hot and humid. It is also the rainy season when many days end with a pretty healthy storm with some good doses of thunder and lightning. But it sure turns everything green! Hurricanes that often work their way through Florida are usually just tropical storms over the mainland. There was a pretty severe tornado several years ago, but it's pretty rare. The sale of weather radios rocketed. Orlando radio stations have excellent coverage when tornado and severe storm watches are in effect.

Here are the Weather Channel's statistics for the winter months:

- January -average high 68, average low, 48, mean 56

- February - average high, 71, average low, 49, mean, 57

- March - average high, 76, average low, 52, mean, 64.

I should also add that The Villages properties are generously adorned with ponds for retaining water. The Villages sheds water like a duck; and even with the strongest downpours, flooding problems are rare.

Volunteering in the Villages

For the most part Villagers are very caring, giving people. Each Sunday in the Villages Daily Sun there is a listing of volunteer opportunities. Here are just a few of the opportunities available:

- o AARP tax aide

- o American Cancer Society

- o Food pantries

- o Libraries

- o Make-A-Wish Foundation

- o Habitat for Humanity

- o Operation Shoebox (one of the largest in the US)

- o Angel Snugs (which recently created their 10,000th hat for children with special needs around the country.

- o Hospice

- o Salvation Army

- o SCORE (Service Core of Retired Executives)

- Honor Flight

- Special Olympics

- And many, many more

Veterans in The Villages

There is a huge concentration of veterans in The Villages (One out of every 5 residents is a veteran). The state of Florida is home to 1.5 million veterans which is the third largest veteran population in the U.S. - and more than half of them are over 65. There are more than 100,000 WW II veterans in Florida - a number that is shrinking all too fast. There are 28 veterans clubs within The Villages including the World War II History Club, Disabled American Veterans Chapter 150, Marine Corps League Detachment No. 1267, Veterans of Foreign Wars Post 1267, Viet Nam Veterans, and Combat Veterans to Careers. Veteran's Day and Memorial Day are celebrated at Veteran's Memorial Park near Spanish Springs. And on these holidays hundreds of Villages homes are decorated with flags - a very moving experience. There is also a Military Retirees Activities Office to help retired veterans with questions concerning benefits and related subjects.

In 2012 a brand new state of the art 99,000 square foot Veterans Outpatient Clinic was opened on the northern border of The Villages to serve vets in the area. There are also large VA Hospitals in Tampa and Gainesville.

The local American Legion Post 347 boasts being the world's largest post with more than 5000 members. It is a very active post with many events and is the starting and ending point for some of the largest Honor Flights. This past spring (2014) I was witness, along with over a thousand others to the return of an Honor Flight of over 50 World War II veterans. The celebration included a number entertainers and musicians from the area who gave of their time to welcome home these brave warriors. When the busses returned they were led by about 40 motorcyclists from the local Nomads. Truly a night to remember!

There is also a very large Operation Shoebox staffed by many Villages volunteers. Their effort is truly remarkable.

The Adopt-A-Bench Program

A very unique program in The Villages that adds beauty to the surroundings while helping people honor their lost ones is called the Adopt-A-Bench Program.

Residents can honor a loved one and clubs and organizations can show their participation in the community by "adopting" benches (The cost is $675.) to be placed throughout The Villages. Each bench features a plaque displaying a personalized message. Many of those who adopt these benches tastefully decorate them for the holidays.

Schools in The Villages

Right about in the geographical center of The Villages on Route 466 are the campuses of The Villages High School, Middle School, and Elementary School. These charter schools are among the most successful in Florida and are available to families of those who are employed by The Villages and businesses that serve The Villages. 99% of the students graduate, and 93% advance to higher education which attests to the quality of education there. These schools have very high quality sports programs with a lot of support from Villages residents.

Churches in The Villages

The fact that The Villages is in the Bible belt is pretty obvious. There are many, many churches in the area many of which have grown to mega-church size. There is also a fairly new Jewish Synagogue adjacent to the property. Churches are very active and, a major section of Saturday's newspaper is devoted to their schedules.

Employment in The Villages

The Villages has created many employment opportunities and for those who seek full or part time work. A good place to start your search is on the website, Careers in the Villages. There you will find careers within The Villages, Villages Community Development District jobs, jobs in the local community, and Charter School employment. Don't expect to get rich with these, since the pay is not that great. The jobless rate in Sumter County is 4.7% compared to 5.4% statewide.

Here are a few facts and statistics that may surprise you:

- The average age in The Villages for a male is 62 and female is 60.

- In 2011, The Villages sold almost one percent of all the new homes in the entire United States.

- The population of the Villages grows by approximately 4,500 annually.

- The Villages population passed 93,000 in 2012 with the total population projected to be close to 110,000 by 2015. An average of 20 people move into The Villages every day.

- One real estate journal reported that The Villages sold about 2.5 times more homes than the second largest development in the United States in 2011.

- To maintain its senior-citizen status under federal law, at least 80 percent of homes must be occupied by at least one person who is 55 years of age or older.

- Forbes Magazine named The Villages as the fastest growing town (under 100,000) in the United States from 2007 to 2010, about 25% more than second fastest Pecos, Texas, and far ahead of the rest in the top 25 fastest.

- There are about 46,000 homes occupied in The Villages as of January 1, 2013. The current projected total number of home sites available at build out is 56,268.

- Persons under the age of 19 years are not permitted to reside within The Villages but may visit for a maximum of 30 days per year unless a longer exemption is granted.

- New Homes sold in the Villages average 200-250 per month.

- Half of the people buying homes in The Villages pay cash for their house.

- The average household income for home buyers in The Villages is $93,800.

- When The Villages opened up home sales South of CR 466A – 55homes sold in first eight days.

- The Villages is planned to be home to 2.7 million square feet of commercial buildings and retail tenants.

- The Villages population is larger than 93.4% of the municipalities in Florida (28th largest of 411).

- The Villages population is larger than 31 of the 67 counties in Florida.

- There are five water towers in The Villages.

- There are over 1,200 miles of water mains. There are over 8,000 manholes in The Villages.

- There are ten commercial areas (Lake Sumter Landing, Spanish Springs, La Plaza Grande, Buffalo Ridge, Colony Plaza, Southern Trace, Spanish Plaines, Mulberry Grove, Brownwood Paddock Square, and soon Antrim Dells (will be next to Brownwood Square).

- At build-out, the population of The Villages will make it the 14th largest municipality in Florida.

- The developer listens to Village residents and consequently the resident survey for 2010 had a 97% satisfaction rating!

- The CBS Sunday Morning segment of May 2011 featured a video segment on The Villages Golf Carts and it continues to make the rounds on YouTube with over 4 million views.

- The Villages is the safest single site development in the country with the lowest crime rate.

- The Villages has seven fire stations. The Villages Public Safety Department has almost 90 employees. About 70% are trained medics and 30% are trained EMT's.

- The Villages Community Watch is comprised of six full time and 294 part time employees. According to the Community Watch, its employees patrol 80,000 miles of neighborhood streets each month while averaging more than 3.5 passes by everyone's home every 24 hrs. In 2011, employees performed more than 209,000 security activities or actions during the year.

- 10,230 calls were made by the Public Safety Department in The Villages in a recent year – about 1% were for fires (flames), 10% were service calls, 9% were false alarms, and 80% were medical/rescue calls.

Chapter 2

Golf, Golf, and More Golf; Sports in The Villages

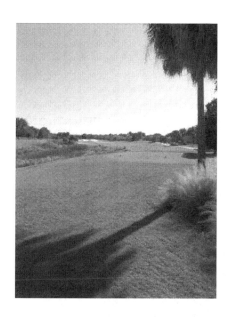

Golf in The Villages

The Villages residents for the most part are very active people. From the very beginning, The Villages has been developed as a golf community. The development of each new village generally begins with the laying out (and sometimes completion) of new executive and championship courses. That is followed by any necessary fire stations and then the pools, mail centers, and recreation centers. Then come the homes, and they are build at an alarming rate. In about the same time as I can build a bird house, the construction crews will build several homes. There is a pretty healthy premium for any who are crazy enough to have a golf course view. Okay, maybe that's not true all the time, but Villages golfers are not generally all known for their accuracy. And some of the golf view homes have golfers closing in on their back yards every few minutes.

Here are a few statistics regarding golf in The Villages that might surprise you:

- The Villages has more holes of golf than any other community/facility in the world, currently at 603 holes. (Mission Hills in China is second with 216 holes).

- That's a total of 96.1 miles, tee to green, which would be about the distance between New York City and Philadelphia!. This means that you could golf 18 holes a day for a month and still not golf every hole!

- At build out, there will be 621 holes of golf in The Villages.

- By final build out, The Villages will operate 12 country-club championship courses.

- There are between 13,800 and 17,600 tee times available each day in The Villages, the higher number being in the summer with the long Florida days.

- A player shooting par golf would have a score of 924 on the Executive Golf trail and 1224 on the championship courses totaling 2148. A bogie shooter would have a total of 2751!

- In a recent year a total of 55,663 Villagers played one or more rounds of golf for a total of 2,546,611 rounds of golf. The approximate number of miles driven in golf carts for this many rounds of golf on The Villages golf courses total 6,330,365 miles. That's a distance equivalent to driving around the world at the Equator 254 times.

- There were 1,832 holes-in-one recorded in The Villages in 2011. That's five holes in one recorded every day of the year in 2011.

- 316 Villagers shot their age or better last year a total of 1,500 times.

- Statistically, there were 5,810,493 golf balls lost in The Villages in a recent year (I, for one, would really like to know how that was determined). We often joke around that ponds in The Villages rise several inches a year from our "sacrificial golf balls).

- About one-third of Villages residents are regular golfers.

- Playing 36 holes per day, a Villager could play 15 straight days of golf in The Villages without repeating a hole.

- 315 Holes of golf in The Villages have received Audubon International's Silver Certified Sanctuary Designation.

You can get detailed information about championship and executive courses at the **Golf in the Villages** website. Here you will find descriptions of all 33 executive courses and 12 championship ones as well as rates, handicaps and other information.

Not all people in The Villages are golfers. It is estimated that one third of the residents play golf regularly. And there are some who golf nearly every day. There is a rather unique golf tee time system that can be accessed either by phone or email. The phone system is a bit cumbersome, so many opt to use thevillages.net to view and schedule tee times. There is a cost of $8 per month for this service. There is a point system that accesses points for each time you play and also penalty points for when you don't show up or cancel. Allowance is given for weather related situations (rain, thunder/lightning, hurricanes, tornados, tsunamis, freezes etc.). It is a very fair system that strives to give residents an equal chance to get tee times. For most of the year it works very well; but in the busy months of January through March, it's a little tougher to get the tee times you want.

Executive course golf is free for all residents as well as those who are renting (as long as the owner temporarily hands in their ID cards). There is a "trail fee" of $4.00 for each player unless they have paid the annual fee of about $140 per couple. Costs of playing the championship courses vary throughout the year, the most expensive being December - April. During these months many Villages opt for the better deals at one of the many fine courses in the area (And there are a lot of these).

I was thinking of adding all these neighboring golf courses here but that might bore all you non-golfers to tears (there all more than 30 on my list). So here is a special free offer for you golfers who might be interested in courses near The Villages. Just send me an email at lindsaycollier@comcast.net and I'll send you my list. This list includes direct links to the websites of all these courses. Courses include the many that are in the close-by cities of Leesburg and Ocala.

There are numerous neighborhood leagues and also men's and women's days where anyone can sign up for shotgun scrambles.

Executive Courses in The Villages include:

- o Amberwood
- o Bacall
- o Bogart
- o Bonita Pass
- o Briarwood
- o Chula Vista
- o Churchill Greens
- o DeLavista
- o El Diablo
- o El Santiago
- o Hawkes Bay

- Heron
- Hill Top
- Mangrove
- Mira Mesa
- Oakleigh
- Palmetto
- Pelican
- Pimlico
- Red Fish Run
- Roosevelt
- Saddlebrook
- Sandhill
- Silver Lake
- Southern Star
- Sweetgum
- Tarpon Boil

- Truman

- Turtle Mound

- Volusia (to open in 2015

- Walnut Grove

- Yankee Clipper

- The last three are in planning and construction stages.

These executive courses vary in difficulty, but most of them are quite challenging with lots of sand, water, grasses, and, of course, the homes and backyards of residents. Many of the greens are large and very challenging as well.

Championship courses (and their opening dates) include:

- Belle Glade - 2014

- Bonifay - 2011

- Cane Garden - 2004

- Evans Prairie - 2012

- Glenview Champions -2000

- Hacienda Hills - 1991

- Havana - 2007

- Lopez Legacy - 2001

- Mallory Hill - 2005

- Orange Blossom Hills - 1985

- Palmer Legends - 2004

- Tierra Del Sol - 1996

So at build out there will be a total of 35 executive courses and 12 championship or some 630 holes of golf! All but two of the championship courses (Blossom Hills and Tierra Del Sol) have 27 holes. Some of the championship nines carry some interesting names. For example, the newest course, Belle Glade, names their nines after Native American Tribes that inhabited Florida before the first Spanish explorers arrived (Tequesta, Seminole, and Calusa). The nines of Nancy Lopez Legacy are named after her three daughters, **Ashley** Meadows, **Erinn** Glen, and **Torri** Pines. Nancy has her home on one of these.

There is also a Villages Golf Academy which offers courses for beginners as well as those who would like to improve their skills. Many retirees take up the game of golf in their golden years. It is so good to see people in their 80's and 90's out on the golf courses (some of them shooting their age). The golf system does a very nice job of helping those who may have handicaps to play their game, enabling carts to approach the holes more closely.

There is also a very popular Golf Fest each year at the Polo Grounds which attracts a pretty big crowd.

Other Sporting Activities in The Villages

Not a golfer? There are so many other choices for any who would like to participate in other sports. Here is a list of some of other sports available.

Archery - There is one archery range at the Paradise Recreation Center in the historic section.

Air Guns

Badminton

Basketball (men and women) These are scheduled using the Charter School facilities and other locations.

Bicycling - There are a lot of bicycling groups as well as a cycling club and it's quite common to see them out touring the roads in an around The Villages.

Billiards - I count 29 billiards clubs in the weekly Recreation News. Most Recreation Centers have very nice billiards rooms which are often quite busy.

Bocce - Most villages have a couple of courts.

Bowling - Bowling is very popular and there are two bowling alleys in the Spanish Springs area with one in the planning stage for Brownwood.

Bungee Jumping (only kidding- but I wouldn't be surprised to see one pop up one of these days

Cricket

Croquet and Lawn Bowling - There is an area set aside near the Rio Grande pool for these British sports. I'm told that membership and whites are required.

Dragon Boating - There are at least 8 Dragon Boat clubs in The Villages.

Dart Baseball - An indoor sport where darts replace bats and no bases are run.

Fencing - En guard! The Lifelong Learning Collage offers a 4-week class, and the club meets twice per week.

Fishing - There are designated ponds for fishing and many of the waterways are restricted. It's catch and release only. However, for the avid fisherman there are many lakes in the area (Remember one of the counties is Lake County). There are actually 165,643 acres of fresh water lakes within 40 minutes of The Villages. I'm not a fishermen but am told that the fishing is great in many of these waterways. And, of course, there is always the Atlantic Ocean and the Gulf about an hour away for some deep sea fishing - and a Deep Sea Fishing Club to boot.

 Golf Bocce - This has recently cropped up as a popular combination of bocce and golf. I'm not sure but it may have been invented by a villager.

Handball

Horseshoes - Every village has a nicely laid out horseshoe area and there are few clubs that gather for these events.

In-Line Skating - Golf trails are a great place for this sport.

Kayaking - Getting quite popular and several times a year there are events to help people get started in the sport.

Lawn Bowling - Like Bocce but uses non perfectly round balls called bowls.

Petanque - This is a French version of bocce with some slightly different rules .

Pickle Ball - This is one of the most popular sports because it is easy to play, fun, and a great social get together. There are probably about 115 pickle ball courts throughout The Villages at this time. This is a miniature game of tennis played with a wooden paddle and a whiffle type of ball. By the way, the story goes that its name comes from the inventor's Golden Retriever, Pickle.

Pilates

Platform Tennis - Seabreeze , Eisenhower, and Rohan Recreation Centers each have six courts and free lessons are provided.

Polo - The Villages has its own Polo stadium (the second largest in the country) and Polo leagues. The Villages polo club has the largest polo crowds in the U.S. with over 30,000 spectators a year. Polo matches in the fall and spring are becoming increasingly popular. There is grandstand viewing, but many spectators line the fields with their golf carts and make a tailgate party of it. People can go out and stomp divots at half time - but you have to watch out for what you stomp!

Quoits

Racquetball - This is a sore spot for me since I love to play this sport and would love to have some courts available. There are no courts but there is a racquetball group that plays several mornings each week in an outdoor court in the town of Lady Lake close by.

Shuffle Ball - Each village has a shuffle ball court.

Soccer - A senior version of soccer is played on 50-yard by 40-yard fields each Friday at the Villages Polo Club. There are no goal keepers or referees and the playing periods are lowered to 10-15 minutes.

Softball - Softball is very popular in The Villages. There are currently 17 softball leagues and three softball complexes, Buffalo Glen, Saddlebrook, and Jon G. Knudson Field. A new one is just being built in the southern sector. To join you must go through three days of evaluations by resident volunteers. Then you are slotted into a league that is the best fit for your playing level. At that point you are eligible to become a roster player or sub. There are currently 133 men's softball teams, 15 ladies teams, and 68 co-ed teams competing in 17 leagues over three seasons. Villagers play 5,200 softball games each year throughout the 3 seasons (winter, spring, and fall).

Spear Throwing - Yes, I'm serious. Where else but in The Villages would you find a spear throwing club?

Stickball - Played at The Villages Regional High School on weekends.

Swimming (including synchronized) - As mentioned earlier there are many swimming pools scattered around The Villages. But there are four sport pools (La Hacienda, Savannah, Laurel Manor, and Lake Miona) that are dedicated to various water sport programs such as water volley ball, laps, and exercise.

Table Tennis - A very active table tennis club plays weekly at the Laurel Manor Recreational Center.

Table Shuffleboard - It's available at the Eisenhower Recreation Center.

Tennis - There are more than 100 courts in The Villages, most of them free for residents. Two country clubs

(Nancy Lopez and Glenview) also have clay courts but are available only to those with priority membership. For those who are experiencing creaky knees, "short court tennis" is gaining in popularity and available at Sterling Heights and Fishhawk Recreation Centers.

Track - Events are held at the Villages Regional High School, includes sprinting, long distance, long jumps, high jumps, javelin, discus, and shot-put.

Volleyball - There is one beach volley ball court in the Sea Breeze Regional Recreation Center. Volleyball for Villagers is also played in the Charter School gym at scheduled times.

Special Sporting Events

The two largest recreation events in The Villages each year are Camp Villages with over 7,000 Villagers and grandchildren participating and the Senior Games where Villagers compete in multiple events in sixteen different sports ranging from bocce to basketball, to archery to volleyball. 1,417 athletes participated in one or more events in this year's Senior Games in The Villages, totaling 2,796 entries in all 16 sports. The Villages also sponsors a Special Olympics each year.

Chapter 3

Clubs in The Villages

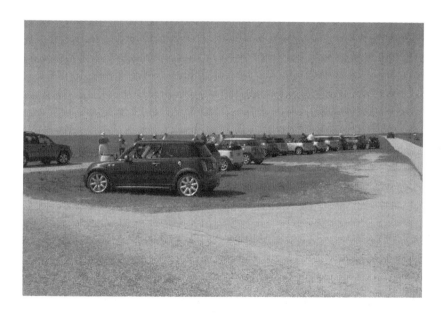

There are over 2200 clubs in The Villages! If you can't find something to do here you have a real problem. The website, VillageActivities.com, does a nice job of listing all the clubs along with appropriate contacts and websites (if they have one). Here is my attempt to classify some of the clubs here in The Villages. In addition, the possibility of beginning a new club is there for anyone.

Music related:

- Classical Music Lovers

- Jazz Lovers and More Jazz

- Dixieland jazz

- Rock and Roll

- Guitar

- Ukulele

- Dulcimer

- Drum Corps

- Bach with a Beat

- Kazoo

- Opera Lovers

- Karaoke

- Harmonica

- Beatlemania

- Doo Wop and Golden Oldies

- Antique Brass

- Country Music

- And More (autoharp, American Bandstand, folk music etc.)

Art:

- Artist Helping Artists

- Watercolor

- Decorative Art

- Chinese Painting

- And Much more! (Artists Helping Artists, One-Stroke, Colored Pencil Painters etc.)

Exercise and Dance:

- ABS Plus
- Accelerated Cardio
- Achieve Better Health
- Ballet
- Ballroom
- Belly Dancing
- Bone Builders
- Cajun/Zydeco
- Clogging
- Hula Hoop Fit and Fun
- Line Dancing (They love their line dancing here)
- Samba
- Tai Chi
- Tap Dance
- Zumba

- And More

Geographical:

- Carolinas
- California
- Cincinnati
- Colorado
- Connecticut
- Erie
- Florida
- Georgia
- Kentucky
- Indiana
- Iowa
- Louisiana
- Maine/Vermont
- Massachusetts - Bay State

- o Michigan

- o Mid Atlantic States

- o New York (Central New York, NYC, Bronx, Saratoga County, Long Island, Buffalo)

- o New Hampshire

- o New Jersey

- o Nova Scotia

- o Ohio

- o Pittsburgh

- o Pennsylvania

- o Rhode island

- o Texas

- o West Virginia

- o And More

Science and Technology;

- o Apple/Mac

- PC
- IPad
- Science and Technology
- Science Topics Club

Military:

- Disabled America Veterans
- Veterans of Foreign Wars
- Vietnam Vets
- Honor Guard
- Marine Corps
- Operation Shoebox
- Honor Flight

Cards and Games:

- Euchre and Bid Euchre
- Backgammon
- Bingo

- Bridge

- Canasta

- Chess

- Cribbage

- Dirty Uno

- Scrabble

- Mexican Train

- Trivia

- Are you smarter than a 5th grader?

- Bunco

- LCR

- Whist

- Mahjong

- And More

Sports:

- Billiards

- Basketball

- Canoe and Kayak

- Scuba Diving

- Darts

- Deep Sea Fishing

- Dragon Boat Racing

- Bocce

- Bocce Golf

- Floor Hockey

- Pickle Ball

- Racquetball

- Karate

- Soccer

- Croquet

- Table Tennis

- In-Line Skating

- NASCAR (there is also a very active NASCAR model race car club that sponsors a race twice per week in the parking lot at Eisenhower recreation Center - a blast to watch!)

- Stickball

- Red Sox Nation, Yankees, NY Giants and More

- Water Aerobics

- Women Fly Fishing

- Zen

Garden and Landscaping:

- Rose Club

- Bonsai

- Daylily

- Landscape Gardens

Auto:

- Mini Cooper- I happen to be a charter member of this club, and we have a blast! We have monthly meetings preceded by dinner at a local restaurant, monthly trips and events ranging from visits to local attractions to overnight trips, and occasional spontaneous excursions. This is true with many of the following clubs as well.

- Camaro

- Miata

- Corvette

- Fiat 500

- Gem Car

- Goldwing Motorcycles

- Motor Racing

- Vintage Car Club - The main sponsor of monthly *Cruise-Ins*

- Antique Car Club of America

- Model T

- Plymouth Prowler

- Convertible

- Toyota Prius

- Mustang

- Tin Lizzies

- Model A Restorers

- Chrysler Sebring/200 Convertible

- Villages Nomads

Writers:

- The Writers League of The Villages

- Children's Book Authors

- Science Fiction

- Creative Writers

- Wanabe Writers

- Writers in Time (Historical novels)

Hobbies:

- Scrapbooking (very popular in The Villages)

- Old Cowboy Movies

- Quilting

- Genealogy

- Woodworkers

- Model Railroaders - Sponsors four major model railroad shows each year which are quite spectacular.

- Rubber Stamping

- Radio Controlled Boats, Yachts, and Race Cars

- Sports Card

- Stamps

Miscellaneous and Off the Wall Cubs:

- Village Idiots (They boast of having no redeeming value at all)

- Golf Cart Drill Team (performs at various events)

- Canine Drill Team (What can I say?)

- Parrot Heads (It's 5 o'clock somewhere - party, party, party)

- Clown Alley

- Laughing Yoga

- Singles (lots of these)

- 2nd Honeymooners (one of the largest clubs in The Villages)

- Gourmet Club

- Red Hats (lots of these)

In addition there are many, many neighborhood social groups that meet in various venues ranging from driveways to homes to recreation centers and pavilions. These groups range from whole villages and villas down to streets and even circles. Many of them provide support and caring for their neighbors who may have certain needs ranging from family loss to sickness to needing help with their computers. As I said before, this is a very caring community of people.

And, **there is never a lack of something to do in The Villages!**

I should also mention that there is a fairly large woodworking shop just adjacent to The Villages proper where residents can go to work on their projects. They are extremely busy prior to the holidays, building toys for tots.

Chapter 4

Eating and Other Forms of Entertainment

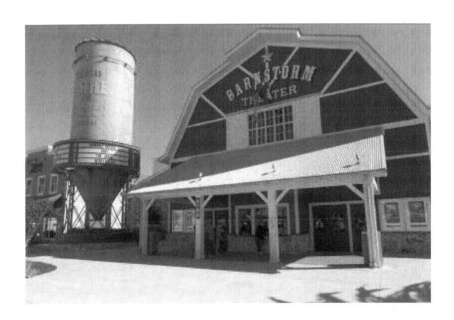

There is always something to do in The Villages. If you want to see all the activities, go to thevillages.com/calendar for a complete calendar of events. Between golf and other sports and activities, most retirees wonder how they ever had time to work. In general Villagers love to eat - and they love to eat out even more. There over 100 dining choices on Villages property and many more nearby. Villagers spend over $200 million dollars annually in eating and drinking establishments! And oh do the folks here love the happy hours offered by most eating establishments! Some restaurants have happy hour all day! And eating out here is usually very reasonable as well.

Dining in The Villages

Pretty much every chain type restaurant has a presence in The Villages. Most of these offer good value and good food. Many say that a lot of these restaurants are a step above those in other locations, because they need to keep up with the quality and value expected by Villagers. Restaurants that don't keep up with these expectations don't last too long here. But where the restaurant business really shines here is with the local ones. The Villages Gourmet Club has a review website that gets more than 9,000 page views per month! Some of the best loved restaurants are those run by the 12 championship golf courses spread throughout The Villages.

- o Orange Blossom Gardens
- o Hacienda Hills
- o Tierra Del Sol
- o Nancy Lopez
- o Glenview
- o Arnold Palmer
- o Cane Garden
- o Mallory Hills
- o Havana
- o Eden Prairie
- o Bonifay
- o Belle Glade

Other notable restaurants within The Villages include:

- o Athens NY Restaurant (Greek/Italian)

- o Ay! Jalisco (Mexican)

- o Bamboo Bistro

- o Beef O'Brady's (Sports Bar)

- o Bravo Pizza

- o Cheng's Chinese & Sushi

- o City Fire (American)

- o Cody's Original Roadhouse(American BBQ)

- o Crispers (Cafe)

- o El Ranchito (Mexican)

- o Evergreen Buffett

- o Fiesta Grande Mexican Grill

- o Flipper's Pizza

- o Gator's Dockside (Sports bar)

- o Giovanni's Ristorante (Italian)

- o Honest John's Whiskey & Provisions

- o Katie Belle's (American)

- o Las Tapas (Spanish)

- o Lighthouse Point (Sports Bar)

- o Li'l Bits (Cafe/Breakfast)

- o Luiginos (Italian)

- o Margarita Republic(Caribbean Sports Bar)

- o McAllister's Deli

- o McCall's Tavern (American BBQ)

- o Mezza Luna (Italian)

- o Moe's Southwest Grill (Mexican)

- o NYPD Pizzeria

- o Oasis Bar and Grill (Cafe)

- o Redsauce (Italian)

- o Ricardi's Italian Table

- o RJ Gators (Sports Bar)

- Sakuri Sushi & Grill (Japanese)

- Scooples Ice Cream Parlor & Restaurant

- Sonny's Real Pit BBG

- Son Rise Cafe (American Cafe)

- Square 1 Burgers

- Steak and Shake

- Thai Ruby

- TooJays Original Gourmet Deli (American Deli)

- VKI Japanese Steakhouse

- Waterfront Inn (American)

- World of Beer (American Brew Pub)

And then there are dozens of fine eating establishments outside the confines of The Villages. But I think you get the point - Eating is an experience here. And, compared to many other parts of the country, it is also a great bargain!

Entertainment on the Town Squares

There are 3 town squares in The Villages - Spanish Springs, Sumter Landing, and Brownwood. Each one has entertainment in the form of a musical group or DJ every night of the year from 5-9 pm. There is plenty of room for dancing, and there are plenty of dancers. And if you are a line dancer you'll be in second heaven! And each square has several bar sites and certain happy hours. You can always tell when happy hour is coming because the lines begin to form. The entertainment is generally quite good and a good mixture of pop, rock, jazz, and country groups or DJ's. There is some wonderful talent in and around The Villages!

There are several parades and festivals during the year to include Oktoberfest, St Patrick's Day, Italian Fest and more. Each year they are decorated with very large Christmas trees with a very festive tree lighting ceremony. Also, there is an annual Christmas parade held at the Polo Grounds in early December which is quite elaborate.

Spanish Springs has vendor's nights on Monday and Wednesday; and Sumter Landing on Tuesday and

Thursday. Brownwood has a Farmers Market on Saturday mornings from 9-1, and Spanish Springs has one on Thursdays. And several times each year there are craft shows at the town squares which are very well attended.

Each year local car clubs have a showing (usually at Sumter Landing). This includes the Mini Cooper, Convertible, Corvette and others. And at Spanish Springs once each month, the Vintage Car Club sponsors a **Cruise In** which sometimes brings in close to 200 cars. Some of the cars that take part in these cruise-ins are simply amazing!

Each town square has a movie complex, and they are all quite unique. The **Rialto** in Spanish Springs and the **Old Mill Playhouse** in Sumter Landing are both very nice and very comfortable. But the **Barnstorm Theater** in Brownwood is the most unique of all. It has to be seen to be believed! A very generous amount of memorabilia of old Florida is used to decorate the lobby area and even the restrooms are uniquely designed to look old. You need to see it to believe it!

 As I mentioned earlier, cameras are mounted in each square and there is a very unique website so you can see what is happening at any time and perhaps wave to your friends as they cuddle around their fireplaces trying to keep warm up north. Please, no mooning! Check it out at Villages Live Cams.

Katie Belles

In Spanish Springs there is Katie Belles which is a restaurant and entertainment venue reserved for Villagers and their guests. They have good food and great entertainment from some of the most talented musicians in the area. Some shows are open and some require tickets, and they are all class acts! A Villages ID or guest pass in needed for entry. Other dining and entertainment venues in The Villages are open to everyone.

 Katie Belles will be closed for the summer of 2015 to undergo a substantial renovation which will involve some rather drastic changes to its interior.

Villages Entertainment Venues

The Sharon Morse Performing Arts Center (referred to as "The Sharon"), located in Spanish Springs, opened in April 2015. This state -of-the-art venue has seating for 1018 people (660 floor seats, 180 mezzanine, and 178 balcony).

The Savannah Center, with seating for about 700, has been the main venue for several years and has provided many absolutely wonderful shows which are offered to Villagers at fairly attractive prices.

The New Covenant United Methodist Church which is just south of Route 466 in the center of The Villages was expanded a few years ago and now provides a new, popular venue for shows.

The entertainment at these venues is always first class. Entertainers like Kenny Rodgers, Bobby Vinton (who lives close by in Ocala), The Fifth Dimension, Willie Nelson, Herman's Hermits with Peter Noone, The Lettermen, Chubby Checker, Melissa Manchester, and Bobby Goldsboro (who lives just north in Ocala) have put on some spectacular shows! I'm amazed at the energy that some of these aging entertainers still have. When Bobby Goldsboro comes to The Villages he also displays his art which is very, very nice.

The entertainment that has surprised us the most are the many tribute bands, some of them that are almost better than the real ones. In the past few years these have included ABAA, the Eagles, the Bee Gees, Chicago, Elton John, Neil Diamond, the Four Seasons, Frank

Sinatra, Bruce Springsteen, Barbara Streisand, Frank Sinatra, and more.

Another popular entertainment venue close to The Villages is the Orange Blossom Opry just a few miles east in the town of Weirsdale. They offer mostly country music but have some golden oldie groups from time to time. It's small, unique, and friendly.

There is a tremendous source of talent in and around The Villages. Musicians, actors, comedians, artists, twirlers, clowns, cheer leaders, dancers, speakers, belly dancers, magicians, and more. And many of them perform for numerous charitable events. As I've mentioned before, Villagers are a very caring lot.

Chapter 5

Florida's Healthiest Home Town

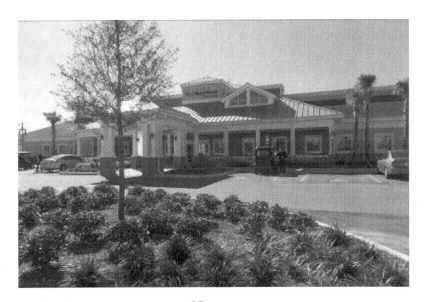

Villagers are generally very physically and mentally active folks. This active Villages lifestyle creates an ideal situation for healthy, long lives. From early sunrise on all over the Villages there are people walking, running, bicycling, swimming and engaging in other activities. And 80 and 90 year olds are out playing golf (some shooting their age).

The survival rate for sudden cardiac arrest in The Villages last year was 44% – about 7 times the national average of only 6%. Average response time to emergencies is said to be less than 4 minutes! Contributing to this high survival rate are the many Villagers taking CPR training – over 7,000 in the last five years and neighborhood CPR/AED programs. More and more neighborhoods are working in conjunction with local fire departments to set up automatic external defibrillators (AED's) at key locations along with trained responders. When a call goes out to 911 the neighbors can quickly react, and a number of lives have been saved because of this.

Let's take a quick look at some of the key aspects of Florida's Healthiest Home Town.

Villages Health Care Centers

For years The Villages has had the motto, "Florida's Friendliest Home Town." A couple of years ago they decided to add "Florida's Healthiest Home Town"' to this and have been working very hard to make this come true. Their goal is to turn health care in The Villages into a *Marcus Welby* approach where patients are treated with caring respect as individuals. So far I believe (from my own experience) it's been a resounding success.

In 2013 through 2014, five health care centers have been opened. These are state of the art health care centers that offer a revolutionary style of care that puts the patient at the center of their own well being. Every doctor has agreed to limit their number of patients so they can get to know them on a personal basis. And each doctor serves as captain of a team of professionals dedicated to the better health of patients. Each facility also has a complete blood testing lab as well as hearing and memory testing. My observation is that the doctors, nurses and professional are very excited and dedicated to this process.

All of these Health Care Centers (with the exception of Belleview) are just a short golf cart ride away, strategically located in Villages locales. The current care centers are:

Belleview - Located in the nearby town of Belleview

Colony - Located close to Colony Plaza on Rt 466A

Creekside - Located near Sumter Landing

Mulberry - Located at the northern edge of The Villages

Pinellas - Located south of Route 466A near Pinellas Plaza

Santa Barbara- Located close to Spanish Springs

They even have their own Villages Health Care YouTube site where various doctors and professionals talk about their ideas on health care.

There is also a unique partnership with the University of South Florida and USF Health which provides a leading edge specialist care center and keeps doctors current with the latest research and medical discoveries.

The Villages Hospital and Moffitt Center

The Villages Regional Hospital (TVRH), part of Central Florida Health Alliance, has been serving patients in Lake, Sumter and Marion Counties for more than 12 years. TVRH has received The Joint Commission's Gold Seal of Approval for healthcare quality and safety in hospitals and was recognized by Modern Healthcare as the fastest growing hospital in the nation in 2012. Their services include premier orthopedic care, interventional cardiology, emergency, neurosurgery and the world-renowned Moffitt Cancer Center.

The new five-story North Tower is scheduled to be finished in February, 2015 and will house additional inpatient and surgical beds as well as a new intensive care unit. The second phase of the expansion, which is scheduled for completion in August 2015, is highly anticipated because it will double the size of the emergency department, add operating rooms and add treatment rooms. The expansion will give TVRH the ability to better serve patients by improving access to healthcare with a total capacity of 323 acute-hospital beds.

Permits have been approved for a second Villages Hospital on 60 acres of land adjacent to Brownwood Town Square.

Other Health Care Services in The Villages and Surrounding Area

There are physicians' offices and special care facilities all over The Villages, and most of these are within golf cart range. Whatever health needs you may have can be taken care of in a nearby facility. This includes a substantial number of urgent care centers at strategic locations. There are a number of very good hospitals within fairly close proximity of The Villages to include.

Munroe Regional Medical Center

Promise Hospital

Leesburg Regional medical Center

Florida Hospital Waterman

Ocala Regional Hospital

And, for veterans, there is a fairly new care facility in The Villages as well as VA Hospitals in Tampa and Gainesville.

Physical Fitness Facilities in The Villages

In chapter two I detailed some of the many sports available in the community to maintain active healthy lifestyles. There are also two fully staffed athletic clubs (MVP), one in Spanish Springs and one in Brownwood. In addition, there are fitness clubs at Laurel Manor, Colony Cottage, and Seabreeze Regional Recreation Centers. Membership is required for their use. And there are also several athletic clubs close by including Anytime Fitness, 24/7 Fitness, Curves, and more. Many of these take part in the Silver Sneakers program through local health care organizations.

Walking and biking are two favorite ways that Villagers maintain their fitness. All the golf cart trails are also used as walking and biking trails. I play in two neighborhood golf leagues, and we are often headed for the courses at 6:45 AM. It is quite common to see walkers and bikers out this early in the morning. There are also two fitness trails with stations for working out different muscle groups (balance beams, sit-up boards etc.) One is at the Lake Miona Recreation Center and the other is the in village of Springdale in the area of the Nancy Lopez Legacy Championship Course.

Most villages have their own swimming pools, and many residents use these daily for their workouts. There are several sport pools that are used almost extensively for planned workout sessions.

In addition, many of the clubs mentioned in Chapter 3 focus on physical workouts through dance and exercise.

Mental Fitness in The Villages

Villagers stay young by maintaining physically active lives. The other key to staying young is maintaining an active mind. There are many activities to choose from in the community.

The Villages operates its own Lifelong Learning College for residents on the high school campus. The Villages Lifelong Learning College offers 2,000 total courses per year and has about 18,000 residents attending around 25,000 sessions each year! The variety of courses is truly amazing! You can see all the course offerings at their website above. Most are taught in small groups (10-25) in Villages Regional High School classrooms. Some take place in local Recreation Centers. Their motto is: "No tests no grades, no pressure - just fun".

About 98% of the instructors are other residents who are offering their expertise. There is just an incredible source of talent and expertise in The Villages. And, of course, those Villagers who are teaching courses are going a long way towards maintaining their own skills and knowledge. Anyone who thinks they may have an interesting course to teach can put in a request through the learning center. They will then carry out a survey to see if there is enough interest in the course and, if the response is good enough, you're in!

Course offerings are quite varied, and here are a few categories:

- Art and Crafts

- Culinary

- Dance

- Exercise and Fitness

- Health and Wellness

- Finance

- Genealogy

- History

- Language

- Music

- Psychology

- Philosophy

- Religion and Spirituality

- Science

- Technology (computers)

- Travel

- World Affairs

They also offer a special speakers series as well as a number of day trips to local attractions. Prices are fairly reasonable for Villages residents. You may also become a patron for $50 per person or $75 per household and receive the lowest course rates.

Support Groups

Based on my own personal experience, an extremely valuable part of health care are support groups. Sometimes there's just nothing better than being with a group of people who are experiencing the same health concerns that you are. Support groups can provide some very powerful healing. When I lost my wife of 40 years to Ovarian Cancer, being a part of a bereavement group saved my life. In The Villages there are support groups for a great many needs to include:

- o AA (There are about 20 of these)

- AL-Anon
- ALS
- Alzheimer's
- Amputees
- Breast Cancer
- Celiac and Gluten Free
- Congestive Heart Failure
- COPD
- Deafness
- Diabetes
- Dialysis
- Hearing Loss
- MS
- Mental Illness
- Overeating
- Osteoporosis
- Parkinson's
- Prostate Cancer
- and More

There are also a number of support groups dealing with bereavement and loss. Some of these are connected with local churches and some are run by local residents. And there is a very active **Shine** (Serving Health Insurance Needs of Elders) group which provides help to residents in choosing health care programs. This is a free program offered through the Florida Department of Elder Affairs. There are almost 30 volunteers who offer their help year round but are most busy during the enrollment season.

Alzheimer's and Hospice Care Facilities

In a retirement community of over 100,000 people, there is an obvious need for memory and end of life care. There are some 21 assisted living facilities within 28 miles of The Villages, most of them offering memory care. At the time of this writing there are several new facilities in the works within The Villages and a number of them in the process of expansion. The Villages Hospice is in the planning process for additional facilities.

Veterans Care

As mentioned earlier, there also is a new Veteran's Outpatient Facility in The Villages as well as VA hospitals in Gainesville and Tampa.

Chapter 6
Plants and Wildlife in The Villages

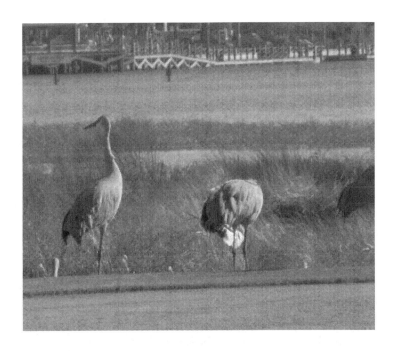

As you travel through the Villages, the one thing that will become obvious is how perfect everything looks. Residents pay a very reasonable amenity fee which covers things like landscaping of Villages properties, golf courses, and water/sewerage. And they do a wonderful job at it. Flowers are plentiful at all roundabouts, intersections, village and villa entrances, and many other areas; and they are pulled out and replaced several times a year to coincide with the seasons. It is rare to see a piece of litter anywhere.

The Villages squares and commercial areas are always pristine and pleasantly landscaped. And the golf courses are all beautifully maintained. I might add that each fall all the golf courses are over seeded with grasses that will stay green during the winter months.

I have never seen an area where so many homes are so well cared for as those in The Villages. It is obvious that residents here take great pride in their homes. Many residents hire one of the many local landscapers, and some (like us) take pride in doing it ourselves. The majority of residents have lawn mowing and care services from one of the many providers.

Most of The Villages property is deed restricted, meaning that there are certain rules you must abide by which results in a very pleasant environment. There are no tool sheds, backyard gyms, fences etc allowed; and fountains, bird baths, statues and the like are only allowed as a part of the landscape gardens in front yards. Architectural approval is needed for home additions, painting etc. These rules may seem somewhat restrictive to some, but it does make a huge difference in the resulting beauty of the homes and surrounding areas.

I don't pretend to be an expert, but I've been a gardener most of my life. Most of it was in New England and Western New York, and there is obviously a big difference between that and Florida. Many plants that are annual up there are perennials down here. And things just grow like mad down here, especially during the summer. Of course there are a lot of things that grow well up north than cannot take the summer heat here in Florida. Hostas are a good example which are very popular up north but, for the most part, won't survive here.

Following are some plants that seem to thrive in The Villages. It is by no means a complete list, but there are lots of nurseries in the area that are much more knowledgeable than I am.

Villages Palms

The Villages location in Central Florida is Zone 9, which means that we are subject to some cold weather and frost. Since a lot of Villagers come from up north, the first thing they want to do is have a yard full of palms. There is a large selection of these, but many of them might not be hardy for the area. Here are a few that are:

Washingtonia - One of the most popular palms in the area and for good reason.

European and Japanese Fan Palms - Japanese fan palm are fast and fat, covering a large area quickly. The European are quite a bit smaller and very attractive.

Sable - Gorgeous and tall!

Sago Palms - Technically theses are Cycads and not palms. Although there are some still thriving here, a blight has taken a severe toll on them recently.

Saw Palmetto - A real native of the area which can be seen growing naturally in local forests.

Silvestri - A fairly slow grower but very nice.

Pindo - Very nice show plant especially as it gathers ferns around its base.

Pygmy Date (Phoenix Roebelinii) - Lots of people here planted these only to learn that they didn't take to hard freezes too well. You're taking a chance but they are very nice.

Bismark- A very different palm and really a stand out.

Queen - Possibly the least expensive and a very fast grower. We planted a $24 special just a few years ago and it's about 60 feet tall now!

Villages Trees

Crape Myrtle - One of the prettiest trees in The Villages during summer months.

Live Oaks - Central Florida is loaded with these stately trees some of which are hundreds of years old. Usually have lots of moss hanging from them and can get rather messy.

Slash Pines - Native to the area and quite beautiful and graceful.

Holley's - Lots of nice choices here.

Monkey Puzzle - I may have the only one in the Villages but it's my favorite.

Bottle Bush - Comes in bush, tree, and weeping tree with lots of bottled shaped flower blooming several times a year.

Magnolia - Good looking trees with nice spring blooms.

Citrus - Fun to grow but a little "iffy" during a freeze.

Villages Shrubs and Grasses

Alamanda - These provides nice yellow flowers but may not survive a hard freeze.

Azaleas - There are so many to choose from and they are very hardy here.

Oleander - These are very popular and fast growing with blossoms on and off during the year, but they can be a bit messy and attract some pretty weird caterpillars.

Camellias - These are spectacular and very hardy. Most of them blossom in January and February but there are exceptions. There is a camellia nursery just north of The

Villages, <u>Bob Wine's Camellia Gardens</u>, that is worth visiting if you want to see an amazing collection.

Bougainvillea - They provide a gorgeous bloom through much of the year but a killing frost will likely end this. The good news is that they are root hardy and will come back strong.

Firethorn Pyracantha - These are very nice bushes with lots of colorful berries that the birds love. It has some pretty nasty thorns though.

Gardenia - The blooms and aroma are wonderful. Ours usually manages to blossom on the day we leave to go north to Rochester.

Hawthorne - This is a good reliable, fairly small accent plant.

Hibiscus - Everyone wants these but only a few of them can take a freeze. Some are root hardy and will come back. It's best to plant in pots that can be brought in during a freeze.

Jasmine - There are several varieties with nice aromatic blossoms - and very hardy.

Honeysuckle - The Florida plants are somewhat different than those in northern climates but are fast growing and very hardy with nice flowers.

Ligustrum - These are the south's answer to northern privets.

Pittosporum - Lots of these were planted by the builders, and they are very hardy.

Roses - Knockout roses do very well all year round without a whole lot of care. Others need a lot of tender loving care but the reward can be quite nice.

Tea Olive - This is a good medium size shrub but don't wait too long for the olives.

Texas sage - These are nice if you want to add a little silver to your landscape. They provide delicate, attractive flowers.

Yesterday, Today and Tomorrow - These are perhaps one of the more interesting bushes with 3 different color blooms.

Yucca - These are very hardy and will give a different look to your landscape.

Bird of Paradise - These are arguably one of the most interesting bloomers.

Chinese Burgundy - These make for nice accent plants.

Plumbago - These plants flourish in many Florida landscapes and show their nice blue flowers during most of the year.

Podocarpus - These make a nice landscape accent plant.

Ginger - The variegated types add some nice color and form but can spread rapidly.

Fountain Grass - There are lots of these grasses in Villages landscapes.

Muhly Grass - I mention this grass because of the beauty it adds in late fall with its purple hue.

Cacti and Succulents - Some are quite hardy in the area and some cannot take the freeze so be careful. They make good potted accents plants though.

Century Plants - These are quite common and hardy but will spread pretty quickly.

Annuals and Perennials

There are much too many of these to mention. But just about all of the annuals grown up north can be grown sometime during the season here. Some will succumb to a freeze and some to the hot summers. Best thing is to watch and see what The Villages landscapers plant along the roads and roundabouts, since they know what they are doing.

I may also mention that orchids do very well here as long as you protect them from freezes. We have beautiful orchids on our lanai, and when we go north in the summer we place them in the shaded side of the house. When we return in the fall we are always pleasantly greeted with new blossoms.

Landscaping Assistance

The Villages is loaded with sources of assistance in gardening matters. There are several gardening clubs, tons of landscapers, loads of master gardeners and the University of Florida Extension Service to provide you all the assistance you need. You can get a lot of very good handouts on various aspects of landscaping at all county offices.

Wildlife in The Villages

The Villages also abounds with wildlife. There are a number of large protected areas that are alive with all sorts of creatures. Of course, alligators seem to interest the most non natives (especially grand children), and can be seen hanging around many of The Villages numerous waterways and ponds. They say that any pond is fair game for an alligator. They rarely bother anyone but sometimes get a little weird during mating season (I used to too). If they threaten any of the residents, they are trapped and removed. We are not always sure what happens to them, but I'm relatively sure the trappers don't take them home as pets. By the way, there are a few restaurants that serve alligator meat which tastes like chicken.

Coyotes, fox, bobcats, wild boars, feral cats, snakes, fisher cats, fox squirrels, monkey squirrels, and rats are spotted from time to time. Monkey squirrels are very different and actually look like little monkeys. They are quite bold, and sometimes they appear in your golf cart looking for snacks when you return from 3 or 4 putting a green. Some bears have been reported in neighboring towns, and one has recently been spotted here. One time while playing golf with my son, a bobcat sauntered across the adjacent tee into the wildlife preserve. And just recently I went out in the early morning to get the newspaper and there was a beautiful red fox in my yard.

The Villages has been an innovator in creating successful, multi-species wildlife mitigation preserves to benefit all wildlife. There are 14 major preserves scattered throughout the area protecting everything from gopher tortoises to burrowing owls to pocket gophers.

There are many birds in the area such as:

- Bald Eagles

- Sandhill Cranes (known here for their wonderful mating dances)

- Heron

- Great White Egrets

- Snowy Egrets

- White Ibis

- Cormorants

- White Pelican

- White Chinese Geese

- Yellow-Rumped Warblers

- Red Wing Blackbirds

- American Coots

- Limpkins

- Hawks

- Owls

- Mocking Birds

- Wood Storks

- Anhingas

- Many Duck Varieties (Merganser, Black-Bellied Whistlers, Eqyptian, etc.)

- Cardinals

- Bluebirds

- Humming Birds

- Sparrows

- Robins

- and many more

Each Christmas season The Villages Birding Club carries out an annual bird count.

Pets in The Villages

The Villages is a very pet friendly place as well. There are several dog parks on Villages property and some outside within easy commute. There are a gazillion dogs here, the majority of them being the small types. Some people here seem to be permanently attached to their dogs. You even see dogs in strollers, a concept I will never quite understand. And, yes, there is even a dog drill team.

Bugs? What Bugs?

Florida seems to have a reputation for being the bug capital of the world. Not true in the Villages, because they can't get Villages ID's. Seriously though, I find bugs to be a much worse problem in New York during the summers. It's rare to see or hear a mosquito here and some say it's because of the Villages insect prevention program. Twice a year for a couple of weeks (spring and fall) the love bugs invade. They are quite harmless although somewhat of a pain in the neck, since you need to remove them from your cars because they will harm the paint.

Fire ants are quite common but controllable. Their stings can be quite severe. And I have heard of some people receiving some nasty spider bites, something to be careful about when gardening. And palmetto bugs can be a problem. They don't bite but are big and ugly and can scare the whatever out of you. There are numerous services available to control bugs.

Chapter 7

Central Florida Day Trips;
Exploring Florida from The Villages

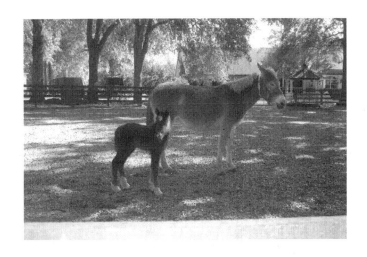

When my wife, Jean, and I first began exploring Florida as a possible retirement place, we looked into the southern gulf area around Naples and Bonita Springs. There are some very beautiful spots down there (Lover's Key and Sanibel Island come to mind). But we found it to be crowded and expensive. The traffic was terrible, and you could starve to death waiting in line at restaurants. Being near the gulf or the ocean may be nice for a while, but we didn't want to spend the rest of our lives being beach bums with little else to do.

The Villages is located in Central Florida between Orlando and Ocala. Orlando and south is flat as a pancake. As you drive north past Howey In The Hills and Clermont, the lay of the land becomes more interesting with some rolling hills. And Ocala has some of the most beautiful horse country you'll ever see. Jean and I are in our ninth year here in The Villages and one of the things we enjoy most is our day trips. There are a lot of things to see that are within an hour or two, and that's what this chapter is all about. One of the problems of living in The Villages is that everything is so nice and there are so many things to do that you don't want to leave. So let's take a look at some of the attractions that will help you get away for a day or two.

Day trips of an hour or so from The Villages

Some of the main destination points within an hour or less from The Villages include Orlando, Tampa, Ocala, and Gainesville along with their many attractions. Some specific attractions for day trips include (in no special order):

Ocala National Forest - The Ocala National Forest is the second largest National Forest in the U.S. and covers approximately 607 square miles of Central Florida. It is located three miles east of Ocala and 16 miles southeast of Gainesville.

The Appleton Museum of Art - A very nice day trip to Ocala if you like art. Stop at Harry's Seafood Bar and Grill in old town Ocala for lunch or dinner.

The Florida Museum of Natural History and the Butterfly Rainforest -About an hour north in Gainesville. While there take a ride through the University of Florida campus. A must stop for lunch or dinner is Satchel's Pizza. This is about the most unique pizza place you will ever see.

Kanapaha Botanical Gardens - A lovely place where you will find the biggest water lilies you've ever seen. About an hour north near Gainesville.

Cedar Key - A quaint little seaside town on the gulf about a 1 1/2 hour northeast of the Villages.

Rainbow Springs State Park - In the town of Dunnellon less than an hour away. While there it may be worth a trip to the coastal town of Yankeetown.

Flea Markets - There are two large flea markets near The Villages. The Market of Marian is the closest and is located just a few miles north on Route 441/27.They have a wonderful selection of fresh fruits and vegetables. Renningers is a bit larger and located about 40 minutes south in Mt Dora. There are a number of smaller ones in the area as well.

Daytona Speedway - For you race fans this is probably a must. Some auto clubs in The Villages occasionally sign up for a tours and a chance to drive the track.

Airboat Rides - There are several air boat rides near The Villages.

Don Garlits Museum of Drag Racing - For the racing enthusiast, this is just 20 minutes or so away from The Villages.

Lakeridge Winery and Vineyards - For some close-by wine tours and tastings as well as a few festivals this is a good choice and only 30 minutes from The Villages.

Whispering Oaks - This opened in 2014 and promises to be a popular spot just a few miles away in the town of Oxford. Their specialty is wine made from blueberries (they have 50,000 bushes). The wine is surprisingly good!

Lake Griffin Park - For a quick getaway this is just a few short miles from The Villages in the town of Fruitland Park.

Half Moon Wildlife Management Area - West of The Villages at 8864 County Road 247 in Lake Panasoftkee just minutes away is what is sometimes called "Sumter's Hidden Gem". This 9500 acre nature area provides for activities to include hiking, horseback riding, fishing, and hunting.

De Leon State Park - Drive a couple of hours, much of it through the Ocala Forest, to this park and have breakfast at the **Old Spanish Sugar Mill Restaurant** where you make your own pancakes at tables with built-in grills. For a different trip back drive south to Deland which has a quaint downtown shopping area. Stetson University is also very nice.

Stetson Mansion - At Christmas time this is quite spectacular and well worth the trip.

New Smyrna Beach - If you are looking for a day at the beach on the ocean side this is a good choice. You can drive onto the beach for a small cost and the town offers some good shopping and restaurants.

EARS - The Endangered Animal Rescue Sanctuary located near in Ocala in Citra spans over 30 acres and exists to provide dignified living for endangered lions, tigers, bears, and more. While in Citra you must visit The Orange Shop for some of the best oranges, jellies, sauces, marinades etc that you'll ever taste.

Micanopy and the Marjorie Rawlings Park - Just south of Gainesville is one of the most natural old Florida towns you'll ever find complete with shops and a couple of restaurants. Each fall they have a very large craft festival which is one of the best I've seen. And the park is just a hop, skip, and jump from there. While in the vicinity lunch or dinner at The Yearling is a must. Don't worry about how it looks from the outside - it's what's inside that counts.

Marjorie Harris Carr Florida Greenway - If you are into hiking or biking this a 110 mile trail that was originally set aside to be Florida's Barge Canal from Palatka on the east side to Yankeetown on the gulf side.

Leu Gardens - This botanical garden in Orlando has a wonderful selection of roses, camellias, and palms and is well worth the visit for the gardener in you.

Tarpon Springs - This Greek sponge diving town on the gulf is well worth a day trip. Shop and dine at the sponge docks, take a boat tour, take the trolley to see all of Tarpon Springs and learn about its history and then, if you have time, visit Sunset Beach.

Pine Island Beach - Due west from The Villages in the town of Spring Hill on the gulf is a neat little island getaway. There is a large Pine Island south of Tampa but this one is small and relatively unknown with a small but very nice beach. While there you might want check out

Weeki Wachee too. The mermaids would like to see you.

Homosassa Springs Wildlife State Park - This is a wonderful place to take your grandchildren. It's about an hour east of The Villages on the gulf and is a sanctuary for birds, alligators, and other wildlife. The big attractions are the manatees with several instructional shows daily about these wonderful creatures.

Bok Tower - This is well worth the 1 1/2 drive south just too see the beauty of the tower and surrounding area and to hear the Carillion concerts.

Florida Carriage Museum - Just a few picturesque minutes from The Villages this museum as a remarkable collection of horse drawn carriages.

Canyons Zip Line and Canopy Tours - Looking for something different and exciting? This is just north of The Villages in Ocala.

Dade Battlefield State Park - Just a short trip south of The Villages is a state park commemorating the Seminole war. There are reenactments every January.

Ocala Horse Country - Want to feel like you are in Kentucky? Ocala has some of the nicest horse farms and is the source for many race horses. Gypsy Gold Farm is particularly interesting because of its wonderfully different Gypsy Vanner horses. They have tours each Wednesday and Saturday.

Lego Land - A bit over an hour south of The Villages in Winter Haven is the world's second largest Lego Land and a good choice for the grandchildren. Years ago this was Cyprus Gardens.

Winter Garden - About an hour away is a quaint (and very affluent) suburb of Orlando with unique shops and a very nice boat tour.

Mount Dora - Less than an hour south of The Villages is the very pleasant town of Mount Dora. There are very nice shops and restaurants and a nice boat trip through Dora Canal where early Tarzan movies were filmed. In October there is a huge craft show there.

Plant City Strawberry Fest - This festival held each year in late February and early March is a very popular event.

Spook Hill in Whales - Probably not worth the drive but if you happen to be in the area of Lake Whales you should check this out.

Fort De Soto Park and Clearwater Beach - These are two good gulf beach choices for one day outings.

Sanford River Cruises - there are several cruises along the St. John's River in Sanford that some of our friends have enjoyed.

Tampa Attractions - Tampa is the home of several worthwhile attractions:

> Busch Gardens - My favorite Florida theme park.

> The Florida Aquarium - Worth a visit.

> Tampa Museum of Art

> Museum of Science and Industry (MOSI)

> The Dali Museum

Orlando Attractions - Orlando is famous for its theme parks and attractions including all of the Disney parks, Sea World, Universal, and so many more If I mentioned all of them I would likely fill another book!

Baseball Spring Training - Spring training is also a popular event in Florida. Check to see where your favorite team plays.

Some longer jaunts and 2 day trips

There are a number of places worth visiting in Florida that more than a couple hours away from The Villages:

St Augustine, the oldest township in the US, is definitely worth an overnight trip. There is so much history, shopping, tours and good food there. And the World Golf Hall of Fame is also close by. There is also the Fountain of Youth for those interested in shaving a few years off their lives. And if you like beaches you'll find some nice ones there too.

Sarasota is full of surprises. About 2 hours south on Route 75, there are some very nice attractions such as the Ringling Museum and the Marie Selby Botanical Gardens. And while there, a drive across the causeway to St Armands Circle should help you to satisfy your shopping needs. From there drive north through Longboat Key, Bradenton Beach and Anna Maria Island.

Cape Canaveral is about a 2 hour drive, and the Kennedy Space Center is well worth a visit. A drive down the coast to Vero Beach might fill out a nice weekend trip. By the way, one of our pass times in the Villages is watching NASA space shots; and we can watch them right in our side yard. It's over 100 miles away but can still be spectacular, especially at night.

The Florida Keys are about four hours south. A pretty dull drive but the Keys are wonderful. Your blood pressure drops about 20% as you leave the mainland. Key West is just a cool and relaxing place to be!

A lot of gambling folks like to go to Biloxi about a seven hour drive. But if you go you are only 90 miles from New Orleans which is wonderful place to visit. But if you'd rather not drive that far, the beaches of the Panhandle are just beautiful. Winter months can be a little chilly though. And you can pass through Apalachicola, a nice little town, on the way.

There are lots more, but that should keep you busy for a while.

There are two books I'd like to suggest if you would like some other ideas of places to see in Florida. **Scenic Driving Florida**, a Falcon Guide by Jan Godown has some interesting scenic drives; and **Weird Florida** by Charlie Carson is a travel guide to Florida's local legends and best kept secrets. I know I've left out a number of possibilities. If there are some you know of that are not here let me know and I'll add them. I can be reached at lindsaycollier@comcast.net.

Chapter 8

Some Closing Thoughts

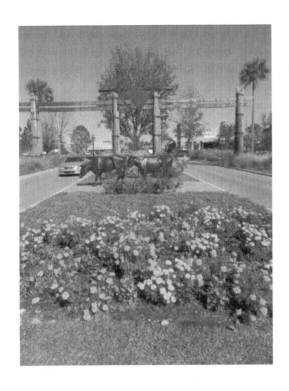

Choosing where you want to spend your retirement years is a big decision. I hope I've painted a pleasant and complete picture of what has to be one of the most complete retirement communities in the word. It is very difficult to think of anything negative about The Villages. One possibility is its size. At build out, there will be well over 100,000 residents. The layout seems to somehow make it smaller than it really is though since most every village has its own identity. The newer villages in the southern sector are all quite large and don't seem to have the charm that the earlier villages have, but this will likely change in time. We've been here for almost 9 years and seen tremendous growth. Each year we ask ourselves, is this place just getting too big?

When we began looking for retirement locations, we pretty much decided that Florida was what we wanted. I have a number of friends who have settled into their retirements in Texas, Las Vegas, Tennessee, the Carolinas and other locations and are quite happy. Some of our friends even decided to live out their retirement in the north. Hey, whatever turns you on! So let me leave you with a few thoughts as to what makes the Villages such a desirable place.

What are the strong points of The Villages?

- Golf cart heaven - give your car a rest

- Great golf, much of it free

- Sparkling clean and gorgeous landscapes

- Wonderful, friendly people

- Incomparable health care facilities

- A plethora of clubs and activities

- Unlimited opportunities for active bodies

- Unlimited opportunities for active minds

- Unlimited opportunities to meet new friends

- Golf cart accessibility to shopping, entertainment, medical facilities etc.

- Great weather- lots of sunshine

- Complete home ownership

- Every service imaginable is available

- Reasonable closeness to two major airports

- Closeness to great theme parks

- Atlantic Ocean and the gulf within a fairly short drive

- Great local restaurants - reasonably priced

- Reasonably priced homes

- Fairly low taxes - especially with homestead act

- Wonderful wildlife

- Terrific place to put your green thumb to work

- Huge opportunity to expand your horizons (physically and mentally)

- Great sunrises and sunsets

- Lots of opportunities for day trips

- Huge variety of entertainment possibilities

- Over 100 restaurants with reasonable prices and, more importantly, generous happy hours

- Lots of people with a great attitude about growing older

What do other residents say?

I could go on forever, but here are what just a few residents say about their retirement in The Villages:

There is only one thing I don't love about living in The Villages. That's trying to explain to family and friends back home how and why this community is so unique. The opportunities to stay well are everywhere: over 2,000 clubs and activities, a well-planned infrastructure of restaurants, shopping and health care, and neighborhoods with activity centers where it doesn't matter what your pre-retirement life was like. We now get to pick and choose how we want to spend our time and our assets. It's a great time in life and a great place to be enjoying it. But they really need to come and experience it for themselves.

Linda Beaulieu, Mission Hills, Bloomfield, NY

You SOULD be interested in The Villages if you want a friendly, warm and established group of ACTIVE seniors surrounding you. We aren't the only place to think about, but we have an attractive, vibrant community of over 100,000 people that is sustainable with a relatively low cost of living. Homes are well built, with reasonable costs and communities are well maintained.

We enjoy practically any type of amenity imaginable. With over 2,000 clubs flourishing in The Villages, your choices range from antique autos to yoga, golf to opera, and computer education to art instruction. But you might prefer your home state club, the polo field cheerleaders, or the happy hour that's everywhere. Town squares are filled with restaurants, dancing, movies and car shows. Lifelong learning activity is extremely high. We are well above average in safety, medical support, and shopping needs or just entertainment. Sports opportunities abound locally while airports, beaches and performing or art exhibits are in easy reach.

Bruce Evans, Village of Chatham, Connecticut and Maine

The Villages is a remarkable place. We enjoy it for lots of reasons and here are a few:

The people are as friendly as they are diverse with folks from all over the country/world representing many different kinds of backgrounds. We have friends from the past (high school chums), from where we lived most of our lives (western NY), and brand new ones (from our neighborhoods and activities).

We golf often, but not seriously, attend various clubs and activities, exercise on our own and at a health club, attend classes at the Learning College, and socialize with our pals. Clubs include; Central NY, Irish American, Greek American, Book Discussion, Liver and Onions, GOFER, Science and Technology, Science Topics, MOAA-Retired Military Officers, and more. We judge at the Charter School Science Fair, help raise money for Wounded Warriors, and Honor Flights for WW II veterans, and do all we can for our neighbors who have needs.

Being able to go everywhere in our golf carts is not only fun but good for the environment. When we do, we are able to appreciate and enjoy the beauty of the forever wild areas, marshes, and golf courses, with the world's most silver-certified Audubon holes (about 600!).

Eating choices seem endless both in and around The Villages. We try to check all of them out, enjoy discovering new places and frequent the best over and over.

133

Life here is a mosaic of good weather, value homes, unending activities and entertainment, perhaps one of the most patriotic communities anywhere, many great friends.....what more can you ask for????

Steve and Kathy Frangos, Village of Bonita, Rochester, NY

I love living in The Villages because of the many activities, clubs and events available to all residents. The active lifestyle keeps us young. Your choices range from golf, tennis, and water aerobics to basket weaving and book clubs. There's something for everyone. Since we have all re-located; we're all looking to meet new friends. It truly is very friendly.
Another feature is the central location. Daytona beach is a short drive to the beach or the famous racetrack. Drive one hour to Orlando and Tampa to enjoy the fun of the amusement parks with visiting family. If you're looking to be active...this is it!

Ginny Fortney, Village of Tall Trees, Oil City, PA and Acworth, GA

I enjoy living in the Villages because of many factors and the top ones are:
*Great people with interesting backgrounds from all over the states and other countries

134

*Super golf courses that are cart accessible
*Many activities and clubs plus the lifelong learning college
*Easy location to both coasts and interesting things to do
*Weather and especially the sun since I come from upstate New York

Chip Wagner, Village of Ashland, Rochester, NY

If you are searching for your own retirement paradise, I hope this has helped; and good luck in your search. If you are already a resident of The Villages, I hope you have discovered some new opportunities. I've done a lot of observing in my 9 years here and a lot of research while putting this little ditty together. But I'm sure I've left some things out. Your feedback and suggestions are always welcomed.

Add Some More

I wish you all a long and happy retirement. You deserve it!

Lindsay Collier

lindsaycollier@comcast.net

You can also find me at Facebook, Linkedin, Twitter, and Google+.

This book is dedicated to the men and women serving in our armed forces around the world as well as our veterans. Being a veteran myself, I have always had a strong feeling of patriotism for my country. Living in The Villages with its extreme appreciation and recognition of veterans has served to strengthen that feeling. The Eisenhower Recreation Center, opened in 2014 is a virtual museum dedicated to veterans.

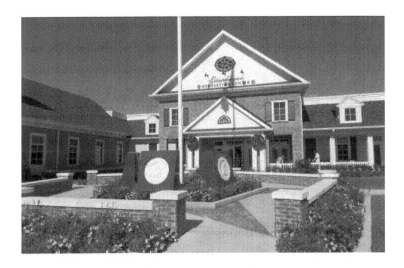

About the Author

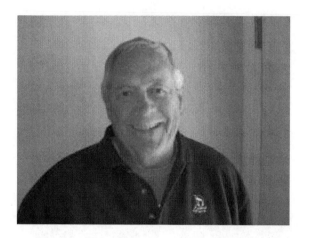

Lindsay Collier presently resides in The Villages, Florida with his wife, Jean. After serving as a Captain in the US Army Corps of Engineers he joined Eastman Kodak as an engineer and took an early retirement after 25 years. During his tenure at Kodak he became their expert in creative thinking and innovation and went on to become an author, speaker and consultant after his retirement. He has shared his ideas with many organizations in the US and abroad in the form of books, workshops, and keynote presentations.

Lindsay is available for speaking engagements on the topic of this booklet as well as a number of other topics. His talks are chock full of great information along with some great humor. He can be contacted at <u>lindsaycollier@comcast.net</u> .

Other books by Lindsay Collier

Amazon.com/author/lindsaycollier

Add Humor To Your Life; Add Life To Your Humor

Organizational Mental Floss; How to Squeeze Your
Organization's Thinking Juices

How To Live Happily Ever After; 12 Things Your Can Do to
Live Forever

Surviving Loss of A Loved One; Jan's Rainbow

Organizational Braindroppings; Musings on Organizational
Breakthrough and Change

Quotations to Tickle Your Brain

The Whack-A-Mole Theory; Creating Breakthrough and
Transformation in Organizations

Get Out of Your thinking Box; 365 Ways to Brighten Your
Life and Enhance Your Creativity

Jan's Rainbow; Stories of Hope

Made in the USA
Middletown, DE
17 May 2017